# THE Fibromyalgia SUPPORTER

## Mark J. Pellegrino, M.D.

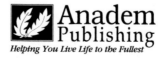

Anadem Publishing
*Helping You Live Life to the Fullest*

Columbus, Ohio

# THE FIBROMYALGIA SUPPORTER

Anadem Publishing, Inc.
Columbus, Ohio 43214
614 • 262 • 2539
800 • 633 • 0055
http://www.anadem.com

Printed in the U.S.A.
ISBN 1-890018-11-2

The material in *The Fibromyalgia Supporter* is presented for informational purposes only. It is not meant to be a substitute for proper medical care by your doctor. You need to consult with your doctor for diagnosis and treatment.

This book is dedicated to my loving wife, Mary Ann.

# Acknowledgements

I have been fortunate to have met many people with fibromyalgia (and their significant others) who have enlightened me and shared their experiences. To all of them, thank you for your help and kindness.

A special thanks to Julie and Brian Hungerman for their help in reviewing the manuscript.

Several people have been especially supportive in my work over the years and of this book in particular, and I wanted to acknowledge their valued help and encouragement:

Ann Evans; a creative, caring and unselfish friend.
Chris and Dave Marschinke; an inspirational and devoted couple who embody the role of Teammates.

# Foreword

When you have fibromyalgia, you want so much to be understood. You want your family to understand; you want your doctor to understand; you want, especially, for your significant other to understand the array of symptoms that especially accentuate your pain. This book does that. This book is for the fibromyalgia sufferer's significant other, the Fibromyalgia Supporter.

If you are familiar with Dr. Pellegrino's books, get ready for another special treat. *The Fibromyalgia Supporter* continues his series on dealing with the pain and debilitation of fibromyalgia. Dr. Pellegrino is unique in how he brings compassion, humor and empathy, then binds it with his expertise to help educate patients. He has dedicated his life to helping others develop positive actions and a healthy outlook toward life with fibromyalgia.

Dr. Pellegrino has been our physician for eight years. In that length of time, we have come to regard him as our friend as well.

You may have noticed that we use the plural possessive case in discussing fibromyalgia. Even though fibromyalgia afflicts only one of us, we are both affected daily by this condition. Dealing with fibromyalgia, like any other illness, is difficult at best, unbearable at worst. The constant pain that no one understands because: "You look fine, how can you be in so much pain?" or "You think you hurt; well, back in my football days. . . (you fill in the blanks!). . ., now that was real pain!!"

It's enough to make you scream, but screaming hurts too much. (We know, we've been there!) Well, you may be alone in the pain, but a knowledgeable and caring supporter can bring a lot of relief to the suffering. This book is a guide for you, the supporter, the spouse, the partner, the caring friend.

This book is about responsibility and partnership. It is easy to be a fibromyalgia supporter, once you understand what is needed. Gaining that understanding can be a long and painful experience for both of you. This book will help shorten that learning period and help you both to a better quality of life. It works!

For this book to be effective, it must be properly applied with love. Noted psychiatrist Karl Meninger once said, "Attitude is more important than facts." This is especially true in dealing with fibromyalgia. The supporter's attitude will rub off on the sufferer - make it the most positive attitude you can. After reading Dr. Pellegrino's newest book, you will be better equipped to help your partner lead the best, most productive life he or she can. You'll both be better for it. We promise! (We *are* there!)

Chris & Dave Marschinke

# Contents

Introduction . . . . . . . . . . . . . . . . . . . . . . .1

The Fibromyalgia Knowledge Test . . . . . .3

1 What is Fibromyalgia? . . . . . . . . . . . . . . .7

2 What is the Pain Like in Fibromyalgia? . .11

3 Fatigue & Fibromyalgia . . . . . . . . . . . . . .17

4 The Brain & Fibromyalgia . . . . . . . . . . .21

5 Wait - There's More to Fibromyalgia? . . .25

6 Diagnosis & Treatment of Fibromyalgia .29

7 What Type of Supporter are You? . . . . .35

8 How to Become a Fibromyalgia
Supporter . . . . . . . . . . . . . . . . . . . . . . .39

9 The Team Scout . . . . . . . . . . . . . . . . . .43

10 The Athletic Trainer . . . . . . . . . . . . . . .49

11 The Referee . . . . . . . . . . . . . . . . . . . . .57

12 Sex & Intimacy in Fibromyalgia . . . . . . .63

13 Becoming Teammates . . . . . . . . . . . . . .67

14 Fibromyalgia Survivor &
Supporter Forever . . . . . . . . . . . . . . . . .73

Index . . . . . . . . . . . . . . . . . . . . . . . . . .77

# Introduction

Somebody you know and care for deeply has fibromyalgia. I have fibromyalgia too, so I know about this painful condition by living with it daily. I am a physician and have seen thousands of patients with fibromyalgia, and have tried to help them learn about it and deal with it in their everyday lives. I have written several books for people with fibromyalgia, but this is the first book for the person without fibromyalgia.

We people with fibromyalgia recognize how difficult and confusing it must be for you without fibromyalgia. You look at us and we look perfectly normal, yet we are always complaining about how bad we feel. You think, "If you look okay, you should feel okay." We think "If you only understood how we felt, and how much it hurts." We might get angry at you at times, but we really do not wish fibromyalgia upon you, although we wouldn't mind if you would borrow it from us for a few days!

You probably have already had numerous articles, magazines, and books on fibromyalgia thrust in your face in the hope that you would read some of it and understand us a little more. Perhaps you have read a little and pretended to understand, or perhaps you just pretended to read a little. Perhaps you found it too complicated or too difficult to relate to since you haven't shared similar experiences. Some of you even get impatient or annoyed.

One of the most frequent complaints I hear from fibromyalgia patients is that their significant other does not support them in their attempts to deal with fibromyalgia. This doesn't mean you don't care; fibromyalgia may be too much of a mystery to you, and you don't know how to support your significant other.

Whatever efforts you have made to become a fibromyalgia supporter are most appreciated, no matter how successful they have been or even if they have not been as successful as hoped up to this point. This book is written especially for you and hopefully will help you learn about fibromyalgia on your terms and at your pace. Heck, you may even want to thrust this book in front of your dear one's face, if it makes you feel any better. If you are one of those people who are still reading up to this point, I don't think you'll be disappointed if you continue reading on.

And remember, reading this book in its entirety will not cause you to develop fibromyalgia or experience any unusual pains. Use caution, however, as you might develop into a well-informed fibromyalgia supporter. You need to consult with your fibromyalgia loved one for proper application of your new-found skills.

# The Fibromyalgia Knowledge Test

Before you read this book, let's find out how much you know about fibromyalgia. To test your Fibro Intelligence, take the following short test and choose one answer for each question. After you are done, look at the scoring section on the next page to see how you fared.

**1) What is fibromyalgia?**
- a) A country in Asia
- b) A medical condition causing excessive hair growth all over the body
- c) A disease of muscle and joints
- d) A syndrome of painful muscles, fatigue, and tender points

**2) Who usually gets fibromyalgia?**
- a) Eskimos
- b) Travelling salesmen
- c) School bus drivers
- d) Women between ages 20 and 50

**3) Which of the following makes one more susceptible to getting fibromyalgia?**
- a) Drinking too much water
- b) Watching TV too closely
- c) Repetitive trauma
- d) A parent with fibromyalgia

**4) What is the key exam finding in fibromyalgia?**
- a) Excessive facial sweating
- b) Detachable teeth
- c) Swollen inflamed joints
- d) Painful tender points

5) **Which is an associated condition seen with fibromyalgia?**
   a) Barking cough
   b) Premature cavities
   c) Scoliosis
   d) Irritable bowel syndrome

6) **What is the diagnostic lab abnormality in fibromyalgia?**
   a) Fragmented pain chromosomes
   b) Undetectable thyroid hormone
   c) High substance P level
   d) There is none

7) **What fibromyalgia doctor specializes in physical medicine and rehabilitation?**
   a) Upholsterers (furniture doctors)
   b) Veterinarians
   c) Rheumatologist
   d) Physiatrist

8) **What class of medicines are used to decrease pain and improve mood in fibromyalgia?**
   a) M & M's
   b) CNN's
   c) NSAID's
   d) SSRI's

9) **What is the cause of fibromyalgia?**
   a) Getting old
   b) Eating too much
   c) Too many whiplash injuries
   d) Don't know exact cause

10) **What is the cure for fibromyalgia?**
   a) Fibrogone nasal spray
   b) Eliminating all foods from diet
   c) Medicines combined with physical therapy
   d) No cure has been found

## SCORING:

For each question, the answers you circled are worth the following points.

 a) 0
 b) 0
 c) 1
 d) 3

For all questions, the correct answer was d. You get partial credit for answer c. Add up the numbers to get your final score and see where you fit.

## Total score:

 **0 - 5**   **Hello? Anybody home?**

 **5 - 13**   **Limited knowledge.** Okay, so you guessed right on a few and perhaps figured out the pattern. You have a lot to learn about fibromyalgia.

 **13 - 19**   **Fair knowledge.** The concept of fibromyalgia is not completely foreign to you and your knowledge is about what would be expected for someone without fibromyalgia, who has a significant other with fibromyalgia.

 **20 - 26**   **Very good knowledge.** You may already be well on your way to becoming a successful fibromyalgia supporter.

 **27 - 30**   **What are you doing reading this book?** This book is for persons without fibromyalgia – not persons with fibromyalgia! Go ahead and read the book anyway, you may learn a thing or two.

Now that you've completed this test, you may put your pencils down and begin reading Chapter 1.

Good luck!

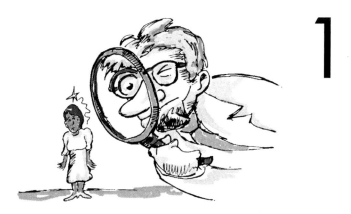

# What is Fibromyalgia?

Fibromyalgia is a common, painful condition of soft tissues, mainly muscles, which causes widespread pain, stiffness, fatigue, and poor sleep, among other symptoms. Painful spots called tender points are found in the muscles of people with fibromyalgia.

Fibromyalgia has been around a long time even though we have only recently begun to better understand and diagnose this condition. Nearly 100 years ago, the medical literature described a condition of "fibrositis" as a cause of low back pain. Inflammation of the fibrous tissue surrounding the muscle was originally blamed for the pain. Medical investigators later showed that there was no actual inflammation and fibrositis became a controversial condition.

Much of the controversy stems from the fact that no specific lab or test can prove or disprove the presence of fibromyalgia. In addition, many doctors did not learn about fibromyalgia in medical school or even believe that it existed.

In the past fifteen to twenty years, however, fibromyalgia has been studied extensively. Fibromyalgia is now well defined using specific criteria. It is indeed a unique medical condition that can be treated even if we don't have a cure yet.

Fibromyalgia is a real condition, causing real pain, even if the person looks normal on the outside. About five percent of the population has fibromyalgia. That means that if you are in a store where one hundred people are shopping, five of those people will have fibromyalgia. Unless, of course, the store is having a special on over-the-counter pain pills, and then you might find that you and the employees are the only ones in the store without fibromyalgia.

Fibromyalgia has been called the invisible condition because you can't look at someone and tell if he or she has fibromyalgia. However, by the time you are done with this book, you may learn some tricks on spotting someone in a crowd with fibromyalgia.

How can we look normal on the outside, but have problems on the inside? You can have the best looking, newest appliance with all the latest technology, but if it is not plugged in, it won't work. Have you ever owned a car that wouldn't run? We're like a car that requires super premium gasoline, but our gas tank is filled with cheap regular gasoline instead. We'll run, but we knock inside a lot.

Here's another way of thinking about fibromyalgia: The tools inside a person with fibromyalgia are defective. The tools are there; they just don't work right. The pliers won't close properly, the hammer's head keeps falling off, the saw blades are too dull, the tips of the screwdrivers are rounded, and the socket wrench is the wrong size. But the tool box looks great!

Obviously our body is a lot more sophisticated, but this is what fibromyalgia acts like. The muscles and nerves are there and may look normal, but they do not work properly. This "malfunction" causes different types of pain, and the pain is not in one area, but everywhere. So when we say those four words "I hurt all over," we mean it!
If you try to fix one area, the other areas will still

cause problems. It's like pain has a constant mass, and if we try to get rid of it from one area of the body, it will always move to a different area and maintain its original mass. So when we say those other four words, "My pain moves around," *we are not crazy!* We simply obey the laws of fibromyalgia physics.

Remember, it is not the outside of the person with fibromyalgia that you care about, it's what is on the inside that counts. That is who you love. In fibromyalgia, it is the inside of the person that counts, because that is where the pain is coming from. We don't need a new tool box or new tools; we need to learn how to get the best use of the tools we have. We could use your help.

We with fibromyalgia recognize that you are also a "victim" of this disorder. Fibromyalgia affects your life, too, and we need to help each other cope with it. So, in this chapter, I have managed to compare your beloved one to appliances, cars, and tools. Unfortunately, the warranty has expired and there is no way to fix our fibromyalgia bodies. Fibromyalgia is a chronic and permanent condition for which there is yet no cure. But we keep looking for one.

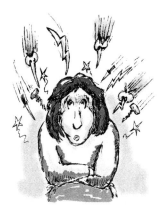

# 2

# What is the Pain Like in Fibromyalgia?

We all know about pain. We've learned from a very early age that pain is a dirty four-letter word.

However, pain is a part of living. We hear about pain every day on TV and learn how bad it is to have pain.

With men, pain is the common denominator that encourages communication and can even be part of the male bonding experience. It is not unusual for men to talk about their painful athletic injuries in detail. Joe says to Jim, "I tore my right knee out in football back in 1974, during the second game against Central, when #68 fell on me." Jim responds by saying "Wow, that must have hurt. It reminds me of the softball tournament in August of 1979, when I was playing left field and lunged for a line drive and pulled my groin." Jim and Joe say "Ooh!" at the same time.

There is your average pain that is part of every day living. You do not expect this pain to interfere with your function. In fact, you may not even consider average pain that you notice after running around or throwing a ball as real pain because it doesn't inter- fere with your activities. If you were a professional athlete you would play (work) with pain all the time. Pain from injuries is different from everyday pain. But even with acute injuries, you have your expectations. One expectation is that your acute pain is temporary, or will disappear over time, or perhaps with medical treatment. Knowing that there is an end point to the pain helps you handle the pain while you have it. You think, "Yeah, it hurts pretty bad, but it will go away."

Another expectation is that the pain will not interfere with your activities. Of course, serious injuries can end a professional athlete's career. But for the everyday person, daily activities and jobs can usually be performed in spite of the acute pain. It is common practice for people to brag about their acute pains on a Monday morning at work. "My arms are killing me, but I put up my son's basketball hoop all by myself this weekend." "Yeah, my legs and back are killing me because I played all the neighbor kids one on one in basketball, and this old man beat every one of them!" Pain can be considered a reward for doing a good job.

We don't think of pain as a physiologic process to warn us that our body tissues may be in danger. Nobody talks about pain as a process that begins at the nerve endings of the skin, muscles, bones or other tissues. Neuroreceptors then detect painful stimulations and neurotransmitters cause tiny electrical currents to travel up the nerves into the spinal cord where the signals are then routed up specific pain tracts to the brain. In fact, Jim would sound pretty silly if he said to Joe "Man, my groin transmitters are really activating my pain tracts." But pain is indeed an uncontrolled physiologic process involving the nerves.

Before I tell you about the pain in fibromyalgia, let me ask you a few questions. What if your pain never went away? What if everything you did caused even more pain? What if your body's physiology was dysfunctional so it continuously signaled pain?

Are those small beads of sweat forming on your forehead? Are you getting a little anxious? I always hear from you how you, too, have everyday aches and pains, so what's the big deal (nervous snicker)? Let me ask you a question from the millions of fibromyalgia sufferers in the world: "Do you really and truly think you know *pain?*"

Fibromyalgia pain falls into that mythical category of "If you haven't experienced it, you couldn't possibly know what it's like." It's sort of like the menstrual cycle and pregnancy things that women talk about.

My fibromyalgia patients who have given birth tell me they'll take pregnancy and labor pains any day over fibromyalgia pain. No matter how acute and severe the labor pains are, the women know that it is only temporary, and that the outcome, a beautiful new baby, is a very rewarding one, in spite of the pain.

Fibromyalgia pain is chronic and unrewarding. There is no end in sight to the pain, and nothing good is expected to come out of this pain. It serves no purpose except to make one hurt.

So, what does it feel like to have fibromyalgia pain? Imagine that you have the flu. You know how your muscles ache all over when you have a flu syndrome. You may become totally incapacitated when you have the flu. You ache all over, you feel sick, and you just stay in bed and moan a lot. Your loved one feeds you, comforts you, and brings you the television remote control when you ask for it. Your flu goes away after a short time and you regain normal capabilities. Once again you can consume large quantities of fast foods, dress yourself, drive road vehicles and return to work.

Now imagine that you have the same flu but it never goes away. You are laying in bed, moaning, asking for another cold beverage, when it dawns on you that you haven't gotten any better. Your doctors tell you that there is nothing wrong and nothing can be done. You hurt wherever you press on your body (and no, your finger isn't broken!) Every muscle in your body hurts, but you still have to get yourself out of bed and go to work. But you don't just do that; you go to work, you clean the garage, you fix the meals, you drive your kids to soccer practice, you pay the bills, and, when you are all done with that, you play a game of pick-up basketball. "Wait!" you say, "How can anyone do that?"

To find the answer, watch your significant other with fibromyalgia. This pain is what people with fibromyalgia go through every single day, and yet they still try to do all of their daily activities in spite of the pain. Fibromyalgia causes chronic pain that is much different from acute pain.

Chronic pain arises from acute pain. In fibromyalgia, the painful tender points are the source of the chronic pain. These tender points can develop in various ways, but the exact mechanisms are not yet completely understood. A trauma, infection, inflammation, or hereditary factors can lead to increased sensitivity to painful signals in the muscles and nerves. Instead of healing or returning to normal after some "insult," these sensitized nerves cause changes in the body's central nervous system. The pain nerves (especially the smaller sympathetic nerves) become more sensitive and hyperexcitable and send out spontaneous painful signals all the time.

Permanent changes occur in the interaction between the nerves, muscles and chemicals in the body causing these painful tender points to appear. From these changes fibromyalgia is born. To summarize in sophisticated scientific terms: the muscles say, "We hurt!"

As if physical pain isn't bad enough, people with fibromyalgia have "other" pains as well. I'm talking about the emotional and psychological pains that come with facing fear, doubt, confusion, stress, grief, guilt, worries and more. There is no place in the mind or body to hide all these pains.

In the final analysis, your pains and our pains are completely different. Despite constant fibromyalgia pain, your significant other is going through each day trying to do everything possible. Give your loved one credit. She/he is strong to be able to go on each day with all that pain.

# 3

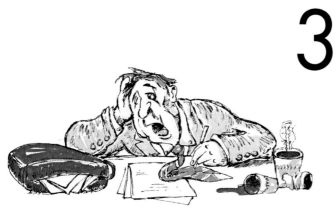

# Fatigue and Fibromyalgia

Next to pain, fatigue is the most common complaint in fibromyalgia. As if it is not enough to hurt all the time, we have to be exhausted as well. Chronic fatigue syndrome is a condition that many physicians feel is very similar to fibromyalgia. In fact, many medical professionals feel that the two "names" are actually the same condition.

Fatigue is responsible for the feeling that your body just runs out of gas. It is why your significant other will say, "I feel like I have no energy to do another thing," or "I'm simply too exhausted to go out," or "I need to lie down and rest my eyes for a few minutes." The person isn't lazy; the body doesn't want to do any more.

The medical definition of fatigue is: "A physical state of discomfort and decreased efficiency from prolonged or excessive exertion, causing loss of power and capacity to respond to stimulation." This definition implies that fatigue is a normal consequence of prolonged or excessive physical stress on normal muscles. Everyone knows what it is like to be "bone-tired."

People with fibromyalgia, however, do not have "normal" muscles, so fatigue has a different meaning. The fibro definition of fatigue is: "A physical and mental state caused when the body's Super Slow Motion Machinery is activated as a result of simple activity, or for no reason whatsoever. This machinery is programmed to run in a continuous mode until reprogrammed or turned off, neither of which is known to occur on a consistent or predictable basis."

There are multiple reasons leading to this definition of fibromyalgia fatigue. Here is a top ten list.

### The top ten reasons why people with fibromyalgia have fatigue:

1) **No Sleep.** People with fibromyalgia do not get good, quality, deep sleep, so energy cannot be restored.

2) **Low ATP.** The body's energy molecules are called ATP (Adenosine Triphosphate), which is stored in our tissues, particularly the muscles. This fuel is low in fibromyalgia.

3) **Autonomic Nervous System Dysfunction.** The small nerves called the autonomic nerves interconnect the major nerves and tissues such as blood vessels, skin and bones and are responsible for keeping the body's internal harmony. Simply stated, these small nerves go crazy in fibromyalgia and use up a lot of energy.

4) **Brain Drain.** There is a mental component to fatigue that causes difficulty with concentration and attention. We become like the absent-minded professor (which is not to be confused with the absence of any mind matter). As you know, we are very intelligent people with a great deal of brain tissue. Part of the cognitive problem is low concentrations of the brain hormone called serotonin, which helps us think clearly when it is in normal concentrations. (See Chapter 4).

**5) Constant pain.** The body's process of monitoring, recording and expressing pain is an energy consuming process.

**6) Depression.** Clinical depression is seen in up to half the people with fibromyalgia and can cause extreme fatigue.

**7) Other associated chronic conditions.** People with fibromyalgia can get other conditions too (see Chapter 6). These other conditions can steal more energy.

**8) Hormonal problems.** Important hormones in regulating the body's metabolism can be low, or inefficient, contributing to fatigue.

**9) Poor use of oxygen.** Muscles in people with fibromyalgia do not use oxygen as well as normal muscles and ultimately result in problems with our energy.

**10) Constant muscle movement.** People with fibromyalgia are shifty characters! That means we shift our bodies around a lot to find a more comfortable position, and have a lot of those habitual movements such as tapping our fingers or crossing our legs, kicking out our legs, or other things that you think we do just to irritate you. We are really doing this to decrease the pain in our muscles. All these extra movements, however, use more energy.

To get an idea of the problem fatigue causes us in our everyday lives, I want you to imagine an energy bank that has $100 worth of energy. Now let's pretend that a normal person (i.e. you) starts each day with $100 of energy deposited into your body's energy bank. As you perform your various daily activities, you spend your energy. More demanding activities cost more. You go through your day, whether it be working, cutting the grass, playing cards, bowling, running an errand, watching TV, whatever it is you do, and at the end of the day you will have used up exactly $100 of energy.

Fortunately, you have normal energy manufacturing machinery, so when you sleep at night, you manufacture another $100 worth of energy to start off your next day.

Now take the person with fibromyalgia. This person starts off the day with only $85 worth of energy. That's because our energy banks have an incompetent administration, a lot of overhead costs, and poor investment returns, so we can't generate the daily balance that we need. Plus, we are required to pay $10 of energy as a daily fee for monitoring our fibromyalgia. Yes, our body charges a very steep security monitoring fee because it is very expensive to watch over all this pain.

Therefore, we only have $75 of energy to get through our $100 day. Are you getting the picture? We have to figure out how to buy $100 worth of energy with only $75 every day. We still need to do all the things that you do, but we simply do not have the energy to do everything. That's the fatigue that we experience in fibromyalgia.

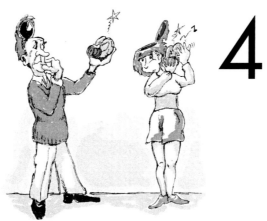

# The Brain and Fibromyalgia

Fibromyalgia involves not just the body, but the brain as well. *Cognition* is the ability of having awareness, knowledge, and judgment to carry out thought processes and understanding. To those of us with fibromyalgia, *cognition* itself is practically a foreign word. We have to read this paragraph three times just to understand it.

With fibromyalgia, our brain does not seem to function properly. We can't remember words or names, and we have difficulty finding the right word to identify or describe something. We are forgetful and absent-minded. We have difficulty concentrating. We have a very poor sense of direction and it is universally known never to ask a person with fibromyalgia for directions to a place. We get our right side and left side mixed up sometimes, or at the very least we have to stop and think which side is our right side before we can figure out which direction is right (or is it left? Did I say that right?)

It's not our fault, but just the fibromyalgia messing with our heads. We even have a term, "fibro-fog" which is used to describe our cognitive difficulties. This fog in our brain seems to slow down and cloud our ability to think thoughts, retrieve memory, form new memory, or be attentive.

A way to describe "fibro-fog" is to imagine that you fell asleep while watching TV. After sleeping for a short while, you suddenly wake up. There is that brief moment where you are somewhat dazed and confused, and you are not sure what time it is, whether it is night or day, or where you are at the moment. This "just-awakened" state of mind clears shortly after you wake up, but during those few seconds you are experiencing our "fibro-fog." Imagine episodes like this that persist for hours at a time and you can get a better understanding what it is like to have fibromyalgia affecting our brain. You can see how we misplace our car keys all the time.

Another cognitive aspect of our fibromyalgia is a somewhat unique personality that we seem to have. People with fibromyalgia tend to be compulsive, highly organized, perfectionistic, time-oriented and anxious. We like to do things ourselves because we know it will get done exactly the way we want it.

Your significant other with fibromyalgia is responsible, timely and reliable because it is too stressful for us not to be that way. You fibromyalgia supporters are usually laid back and not bothered by all the little details that drive us nuts. Sometimes the mere fact that you are able to be like that irritates us!

We can't help the way we are, and it is easy for us to rationalize that our way is the right way. Most of us with fibromyalgia will gladly trade off some of our compulsive personality traits so we could try to be more relaxed and less anxious. We must find ways to see the positive aspects of our personalities, rather than the negative. This is where you can help.

Why do people with fibromyalgia have these cognitive differences? Part of the problem is the decreased levels of certain hormones in the brain. Serotonin is low in fibromyalgia patients, and this particular hormone is responsible for decreasing pain signals in the brain, improving our mood, improving our outlook, and increasing our ability to concentrate. In fibromyalgia, it is like someone turned down the "brightness switch" on our brain TV.

Another hormone that is found in lower concentrations is norepinephrine. This hormone has various duties including enhancing our awareness and focusing abilities, and putting the brain function systems in the "alert" mode. Norepinephrine correlates with the "contrast switch" on your brain TV, and it is also turned down in fibromyalgia.

Studies have shown other brain differences in persons with fibromyalgia. The hypothalamus is a key portion of the brain that controls and integrates a lot of the hormonal and nervous system activities in the body. These include controlling our body temperature, digestion, sleep, heart rate and blood pressure. The hypothalamus may be dysfunctional in persons with fibromyalgia.

Another brain structure, the limbic system, is the center of emotions and behaviors. In people with fibromyalgia, the limbic system may have some changes causing us to react to pain differently.

Another brain difference between men and women is that women have bigger corpus callosums. "Wait a minute," you say "I want to have a bigger corpus callosum . . . Exactly what is a corpus callosum?" The corpus callosum is the part of the brain that connects the right and left halves of the brain. Studies have shown that women tend to have a bigger corpus callosum, which means that the two halves of the brain are better connected and both sides of the brain work simultaneously. Men, on the other hand, have smaller corpus callosums, and tend to use only one side of the brain at a time.

This difference allows women to incorporate more information simultaneously when solving a problem. Women are more apt to use past experiences, emotions, and other broader reaching factors along with the reasoning and action parts of the brain when trying to find solutions to problems. Men, on the other hand, tend to use the action and reasoning part of their brains and quickly address a problem, but perhaps in a less thorough and comprehensive manner. (This doesn't mean that we men are only half-brained!)

Our female counterparts have often accused us of being half-witted or half-brained, and now they have corpus callosum studies to support their statements. Since women make up the majority of people who have fibromyalgia, there may be a price to pay for being "full-brained." Their ability to incorporate all their symptoms and thoughts simultaneously probably play a role in why they are more "brain vulnerable" to having a painful condition such as fibromyalgia.

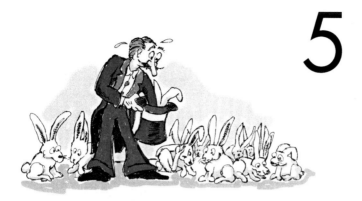

# Wait – There's More to Fibromyalgia?

We have discussed some of the major symptoms of fibromyalgia, including pain, fatigue, and cognitive dysfunction. Believe it or not, these are only a few of the conditions seen with fibromyalgia. Fibromyalgia is a broader condition that involves almost every part of the body.

The following are various conditions frequently seen with fibromyalgia:

Allergies

Anxiety disorder and panic attacks

Depression (can be seen in half of patients)

Dry eyes

Headaches (tension, migraine or both)

Irritable bowel syndrome (diarrhea, constipation, stomach cramps)

Irritable bladder (constant urge to urinate)

Mitral valve prolapse (bulging of one of the heart valves during the heartbeat)

Chest pain

Dizziness

Sleep disturbance (poor quality sleep)

Restless legs (nighttime leg cramps and restlessness)

TMJ dysfunction (jaw pain)

There are a lot more, but I wanted this book to be light enough to carry.

Each of these associated conditions may be severe enough to require its own separate treatment, in addition to the treatment of the overall fibromyalgia. All of these conditions, by themselves, do not indicate fibromyalgia, but if one has fibromyalgia with the typical pain and tender points, these associated conditions are commonly seen. It is not surprising that people with fibromyalgia may be considered hypochondriacs by unknowledgeable people because of all the complaints. But these complaints and conditions are legitimate.

These associated conditions can present their own set of unique problems. For example, say you and your significant other are invited to a party. Because of poor sleep and fatigue, it takes the fibromyalgia person all day to prepare for the party. Once at the party, the smoke bothers the dry eyes and headaches may occur. The fibromyalgia person decides to try some of the appetizers and mingles with the crowd. Just when everything feels a little more "normal" ... what is that feeling? The irritable bowel decides to kick in and scream for attention, and the bathroom becomes the life of the party.

Fortunately, despite all of its problems, fibromyalgia does not progress into a deforming or paralyzing disease. It is not a form of cancer, nor is it life-threatening. It is a frightening condition, though, especially when new symptoms occur. You feel as if you have no control over what's happening to your body or your life.

A common consequence of fibromyalgia that is upsetting and depressing is weight gain. There are numerous reasons for this weight gain, including:

1. Side effects of certain medicines used to treat fibromyalgia which cause fluid retention or weight gain.

2. Decreased metabolism in fibromyalgia due to hormonal factors or medicines.

3. Decreased activity because of pain and fatigue.

The fibromyalgia appears to alter the body's biochemistry and metabolism to slow down its calorie burn-off. Weight gain occurs even if the actual amount of food eaten does not change.

You need to remember that this is still the same person that you love, even if there is more of this person. Your significant other is usually very concerned about the extra weight gain and is working hard to take it off. So in the meantime you can help by reassuring your significant other of the positive attributes rather than any shortcomings of the body.

When you put all this together, fibromyalgia is a condition that interferes with everything in your significant other's life. Physical effects include decreased ability to perform housework, work a job, do yard activities, or just simply get from one place to the other.

Mental effects include anxiety, stress, and the cognitive problems we talked about. There is a sense of being overwhelmed. Emotional effects are anger, depression, and frustration. A chronically painful problem will affect every aspect of one's life. In the case of fibromyalgia, it is not just one person's life, but two, the person with the condition, and you, the significant other support person.

Fibromyalgia causes a constant level of pain. There is a baseline level of pain that is sort of like a low grade flu syndrome that is always there. However, this pain does not stay constant. It frequently flares up and anything can aggravate it, including daily activities, but especially any unusual activities such as doing some extra yard work or heavy housecleaning or playing a recreational sport.

Weather changes can affect the pain. Cold and damp weather are particular enemies of someone with fibromyalgia, as these weather conditions wreak havoc on the baseline level of pain.

Anything that increases stress will also increase the pain and cause a flare-up. Everyday stress does not cause the condition, but once fibromyalgia is present, stress will aggravate it.

Life, by definition, is stressful. I think everyone lives a stressful life, but not everyone develops fibromyalgia.

Even though we do not know the exact cause of fibromyalgia, we know a lot about it, and we certainly know that it exists and is a very real and painful condition. There are many, many conditions in medicine that we diagnose and treat even though we do not know the exact cause.

We are trying to figure out the exact mechanisms and how all the associated conditions fit into this big picture. We have a lot of pieces of the puzzle, but we still don't have the whole puzzle solved. In the meantime, let's all work together to minimize the effects of fibromyalgia in all aspects of a person's life.

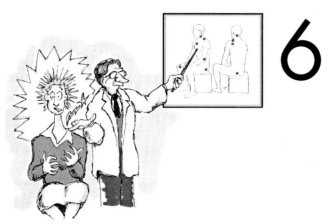

6

# Diagnosis and Treatment of Fibromyalgia

Fibromyalgia needs to be officially diagnosed by a doctor who knows about this condition. Even though a person may have numerous symptoms suggestive of fibromyalgia, medical confirmation is necessary. The doctor will evaluate someone and review the complaints and the nature of the pain, and then will examine the person and may order specific diagnostic tests. All of the clinical information is put together to come up with the best diagnosis.

When I see someone who thinks they may have fibromyalgia, I listen for two key four-word phrases: "I hurt all over" and "my pain moves around." These complaints usually indicate fibromyalgia is present, but the doctor still can't make the diagnosis just on the presence of generalized pain and traveling pain.

Many other people will report that they have read a book or article on fibromyalgia, and after reading it, experience something like a revelation. They may feel, "That's me, this book was written for me!" I would say that nine times out of ten times a person who has read a lot about fibromyalgia and feels that it fits him or her is usually right about actually having the diagnosis of fibromyalgia.

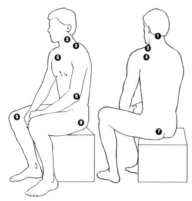

The 18 tender points in fibromyalgia.

The physical examination is performed to look for the characteristic tender points. A *tender point* is a distinct area of muscle tissue that is very painful when pressed on or palpated. A major study done in 1990 found that people with fibromyalgia have 18 characteristic or signature tender point locations in their body, and at least 11 of these 18 should be positive (see diagram). That is, when the doctor with special training presses on or palpates these signature tender points, at least 11 of 18 should be consistently painful. This pattern of tender points is unique and enables us to diagnose fibromyalgia.

A person can still have fibromyalgia with fewer than 11 of 18 tender points, but most people who have generalized fibromyalgia will have at least 11 of 18. Many people have a "perfect" score, 18 of 18 tender points.

There are often spasms that can be felt in the muscles on the physical exam. Some muscles have a lumpy, bumpy nature to them. Normal muscle has a texture of firm gelatin. Imagine that you take this firm gelatin and put some grapes and stands of carrots and a couple chunks of pineapple, and when you palpate this gelatin fruit salad, you can imagine the lumpy, bumpy consistency, and strands or ropy consistency that's present in the gelatin; that's what the fibromyalgia muscles feel like. Check it out on your

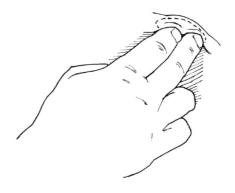

Nodules or ropiness felt in fibromyalgia muscles.

significant other; go ahead and feel the muscles. *Ask first, though, and be gentle.*

These localized spasms or nodules or ropiness in the muscle are very painful, especially when pressed on. The physical exam will not reveal any bad neurologic findings such as loss of reflexes or pinched nerves even though numbness and weakness are common complaints in fibromyalgia.

Joint problems such as inflammation, redness or heat are not symptomatic of fibromyalgia even though the joints hurt. If these abnormalities are present, then something other than fibromyalgia has to be present as well. Fibromyalgia mainly causes the painful tender points and localized muscle spasms.

The diagnosis of fibromyalgia can be made based on the history and physical exam alone, but many doctors will order some diagnostic studies that might include laboratory studies, and X-rays, to make sure that something else is not being missed.

There is no single testing procedure that is diagnostic of fibromyalgia. In fact, routine labs and other tests are normal in fibromyalgia. There are specialized tests on which fibromyalgia patients test positive, but these tests are not considered routine and are often done only in specialized labs or centers.

Just because routine tests may be normal does not mean that there are no abnormalities that can be measured in fibromyalgia. Abnormal tests found in fibromyalgia include low levels of serotonin and norepinephrine (brain hormones) and high levels of Substance P (spinal cord hormones, think "P" for Pain). These are abnormalities in the hormone and neurotransmitter systems that lead to increased pain.

Sleep studies have also been found to be abnormal in most people with fibromyalgia. Tilt table testings show abnormalities where the individual's blood pressure drops when going from a lying down position to an upright position, an indication that the small nerves in the body are dysfunctional. Muscle studies have revealed abnormalities in the oxygen availability, the energy level, and other biochemical abnormalities.

However, there is not one single test abnormality that has been identified by the medical community as the diagnostic abnormality indicating fibromyalgia, and only fibromyalgia. We hope that further research will someday identify a single test to diagnose fibromyalgia, but for now it's primarily a clinical diagnosis based on the history and physical examination.

There is no cure yet for fibromyalgia, but that doesn't mean there are no treatments. The main treatment goal is to decrease the pain to as low a level as possible and try to get the fibromyalgia to go into a quiet or latent state. Even though we cannot cure fibromyalgia yet, we can do a lot to "heal" it so it is in remission.

A variety of treatment approaches exist. I have found that using different treatments from different directions works best. I call it "the full court press." If you are a basketball fan, you know that the full court press is an attack style defense. The goal is to put a lot of pressure on the ball (fibromyalgia) and try to find an opening to exploit. It requires a team effort. This analogy applies to fibromyalgia.

The full court press includes education, medication, nutritional strategies, therapies, relaxation, adjustments, massage, exercise and more. Some or all of the treatments may be needed. I usually try to use a variety of measures at first to try to get the pain to calm down. The patient and I then adjust the treatments to get to the most effective results with the least amount of treatment.

There are really three main goals in the treatment of fibromyalgia.

**1) Learn everything possible about fibromyalgia.** The more a person understands the condition, the less frightening it is, and the easier it is to accept the condition and do something about it.

**2) Find out what works.** What works for one person may not even help another person. Everyone with fibromyalgia has an individual response to treatments and we need to find out what works for each individual.

**3) Establish a home program.** The person with fibromyalgia has to live with fibromyalgia every day, so it is crucial that this person learn how to do any successful techniques on his or her own. For example, if the person finds moist heat, stretching, and an exercise program works well as part of therapy, we would teach the person how to use a moist heating pad, do stretches at home and do a regular walking program as part of a daily home program. That way a person can still be receiving "therapy" even though the supervised therapy programs have been completed.

Hopefully there will be some success with the treatment program, but it doesn't mean the fibromyalgia has disappeared. It is still very much an every day part of your loved one, as it is a chronic and permanent condition.

There are a lot of bumps and potholes on the fibromyalgia highway. We try to teach the patient to find the best car, the best gasoline and the best tires, and to try to ensure the smoothest ride, but there are rough spots along the way. (There I go again, comparing your loved one to machinery.)

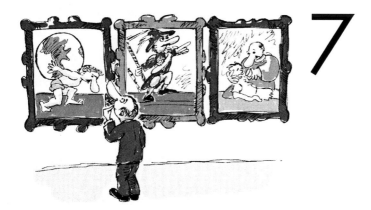

# What Type of Supporter are You?

I heard a joke recently: A woman accompanied her husband to the doctor's office. After his check up the doctor called the wife into the office alone. He said, "If you don't do the following, your husband will surely die:

1. Each morning fix him a healthy breakfast.
2. Be pleasant and make sure he is in a good mood.
3. For lunch, make him a nutritious meal.
4. For dinner, prepare him an especially nice meal.
5. Don't burden him with chores, as he probably had a hard day.
6. And most importantly, have sex with him several times a week and satisfy his every whim."

On the way home, the husband anxiously asked his wife what the doctor had said to her. "You're going to die." she replied!

All the women in my office think this joke is hilarious. After I laughed at it, I thought how this joke is a good example of what it may be like when you first hear about all the terrible things fibromyalgia can do to your significant other, and what changes you may have to make. Fibromyalgia is not fatal, but it can be a threat to your happiness and your relationship. It can be scary facing a chronic illness.

You have an opportunity to become a fibromyalgia supporter, if you want. Then you two can face the scary illness together.

The fibromyalgia supporter can be anybody, but is usually a male between the ages of 25 and 60. Fibromyalgia supporters come from various backgrounds and occupations, and are bonded by a single common factor: They each love a person who has fibromyalgia.

Every supporter is different. Every relationship is different and, invariably, fibromyalgia causes stress which can lead to unique tensions. The main goal is to prevent a strained relationship from becoming a failed relationship.

I have identified six types of fibromyalgia supporters and can compare them to various sports figures. (No, I'm not calling you an athletic supporter!). I use sports figures in this book because I like sports, and hopefully everyone can relate to these comparisons, even if one does not care for sports. To find out what type of fibromyalgia supporter you are now, read the following scouting report.

### 1) Free agent (invisible supporter)

This type of supporter asks the basic question "What's in it for me?" The free agent takes a selfish approach and sees the problem as *someone else's* problem and says, "I'm going to look elsewhere for a better market." Not only is the invisible supporter not involved, but also not reading this book!

### 2) Aging star (disassociated supporter)

This person knows that something is wrong but doesn't want to believe there is a serious problem, so pretends there is no serious problem and hopes it will go away. The aging star worries about diminishing skills and finds it very difficult to deal with any new challenge. The reality of a chronic and serious health problem may be too much, so denial is a coping mechanism. The disassociated supporter wants a quick cure so that things will be like the good ole' times.

### 3) Fair weather fan (impatient supporter)

This supporter recognizes that there is a problem and even tries to understand some of the basics, but the expectations are unrealistic. The fair weather fan wants continuous positive and successful results to treatments and medicines, and is easily disappointed when the outcomes are negative. When things are going well, the impatient supporter is happy, but during bad times, there can be a lot of frustration, negative thinking, and lack of support. The fair weather fan expects the person with fibromyalgia to always be a "winner."

### 4) Rookie (over-eager supporter)

The rookie is eager to please and tries very hard. The skills are there but the confidence needs more work. The over-eager supporter has a hard time enjoying the good times because of worries, fears and insecurities about possible bad times. This type of supporter has a lot of potential that can be developed.

### 5) Coach (encouraging supporter)

This type of supporter encourages the best possible performance from the person with fibromyalgia. The coach puts all the positives together and works hard, studies fibromyalgia, and "recruits" new strategies. The encouraging supporter can criticize, however, and tries to be in control, which includes always trying to improve something, or make it better. This type of supporter does not fully accept fibromyalgia because there is always that uncontrolled element that is chronic, can't be controlled, in spite of the best coaching attempts.

### 6. Teammate (accepting supporter)

This type of supporter is an ideal partner. The teammate is secure and accepts the fibromyalgia. The teammates are playing the game together to "win." The accepting supporter is very open to communication on how to improve, and the supporter and fibromyalgia person complement each other; the good aspects work together for an even better outcome, and the accepting supporter offsets the bad aspects by providing the needed help.

If you can identify what category you fit into, you can ask yourself a question: Do you want to do better? The individual supporter can move through different levels of these support figures. Even if you are already a teammate, you can be a better teammate. If you want to do better, read on. If not, stop reading, but there are no refunds!

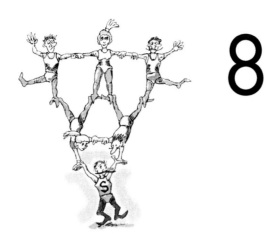

8

# How to Become a Fibromyalgia Supporter

The first step to becoming a fibromyalgia supporter is recognizing some important facts. The following facts are supposed to relieve some of the pressure on you, but also set the framework for realistic expectations on being a supporter.

Here are the facts:

## 1) You are not responsible for your significant other's fibromyalgia.

Fibromyalgia is an equal opportunity disease. It occurs in all kinds of people: women, men, children. It is heedless of age, race, and physical condition. There may be a hereditary susceptibility to getting fibromyalgia, but it is not caused by age, being overweight, or too little activity. Nor did you say something or do something that caused your significant other's fibromyalgia.

## 2) You can't cure the fibromyalgia.

No one can yet. We hope to find a cure soon, but as of now, there is no magic pill, surgery or therapy to completely eliminate fibromyalgia. Fibromyalgia is a chronic condition.

### 3) You do not cause flare-ups of fibromyalgia.

Flare-ups are part of fibromyalgia. Flare-ups can be from increased physical activity, increased stress, weather changes, an infection, or may simply occur without any identified cause. Flare-ups will occur even if all the right things are done, and flare-ups will occur even if you are not there!

### 4) Fibromyalgia is not a punishment, for you or for your loved one.

Are you kidding? We all recognize that fibromyalgia affects both of you, not just the person with it. Your significant other doesn't want fibromyalgia any more than you want your significant other to have it. Your significant other feels guilty enough about being sick and possibly neglecting your needs.

### 5) You can help heal fibromyalgia.

Even if there is no cure yet, a lot can be done to help your significant other do better with fibromyalgia, to heal. Your role is a vital one.

Remember these five facts and you've won half the battle. Now you need to determine how you are going to become a supporter. To be a good supporter, you have to learn how to deal with fibromyalgia. Fibromyalgia is a challenging sport and you have to learn to play the game. That is, you have to become a sport professional.

You are probably thinking that I'm doing it again. I'm comparing fibromyalgia to something else, only this time it's not an object, but a game. Plus, I've given you a new title as a Sport Professional. I shouldn't have called you that, I'm sorry. What I meant to say was you need to become several Sport Professionals, a team scout, an athletic trainer, and a referee.

Historically, men have always been sport profession-als. Early man was a hunter, the first Sport Professional. It was early man's role to venture into the dangerous wild to hunt for food, whether it be in the freezing winter or under the hot, baking sun.

These biologically determined early roles have evolved into the modern male sports professionals, the team scout, the athletic trainer, and the referee. Since men comprise the majority of the fibromyalgia supporters, they are being asked to call upon their biologic instincts, only this time fibromyalgia is the beast.

For you women out there whose significant others are the ones with fibromyalgia, it is time for you to become a sport professional, also. The fibromyalgia is just as much a challenge to the female supporter as to the male supporter, so both sexes can learn to con-quer this challenge.

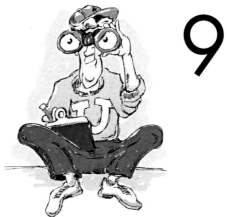

# The Team Scout

The team scout is responsible for gathering as much useful information as possible to help prepare for the game.

The team scout needs to learn about fibromyalgia and how it interferes with function. You know how the doctor diagnoses fibromyalgia, but how can you spot it? What does the pain look like? You need to use all of your senses to spot general and specific clues about fibromyalgia. Pay attention to the details.

How do you put all of your senses to work?

1) **Visual sense.** Look for the telltale signs of someone in pain. You will notice frequent shifting of positions, squirming, or restlessness. Notice that the legs may be in constant motion and can never keep still (you may even notice that this leg kicks you in the middle of the night). Another telltale sign is a person rubbing or massaging the neck. You may notice grimacing when the person does some "benign" activity such as bending over to pick up a Kleenex off the floor.

   Inappropriate clothing, such as wearing a turtleneck sweater in the summertime or a neck scarf at the beach are fairly obvious visual signs.

Comfortable shoe wear may give the appearance that we are "athletic." (Ha!)

A more subtle sight is the presence of goose bumps on the legs of someone with fibromyalgia. This is particularly evident in the presence of air conditioning, when going from a warmer environment to a cooler one, or if there is sudden increased pain or a hot flash. These little goose bumps can be seen if you look closely. (I don't recommend looking too close at a stranger's legs, however, as you could get arrested.)

You can spot fibromyalgia in a second in a restaurant. People with fibromyalgia and irritable bowel problems never eat salads, fried food, or raw veggies. If you see someone with tea and saltine crackers, think fibromyalgia.

You can spot them quickly in a store. Fibromyalgia women are the ones whose significant others are carrying the packages, pushing the cart, and holding the purses. Don't be embarrassed, guys. Your fibromyalgia wives are so conscious about how you'll look carrying their purse that they'll make sure their purses match your clothes.

The eyes are a great visual source of information. Learn to read the eyes. When the mouth responds, "I'm fine," see what the eyes are really saying.

**2) Hearing sense.** If you ever hear the words "I hurt all over," you have audibly recognized fibromyalgia. Frequent and chronic complaints about the weather are also obvious indications of pain. If you hear any of the following: Moaning, groaning, whining, complaining, grieving, lamenting, crying, sighing, or other audible negatives, think fibromyalgia.

**3) Smelling sense.** The sharp biting smell of menthol from a medicated lotion smeared all over the muscles is a giveaway smell of someone who is in pain. For those who are nasally astute, the piquant smell of soapy skin is a good clue that this person takes frequent hot showers.

The absence of smell is also an important clue. Since most strong odors of cologne and perfume make people with fibromyalgia want to gag and upchuck, these are almost never used. So if you aren't smelling anything, think fibromyalgia, but try not to psychoanalyze this too much.

**4) Touch sense.** Fibromyalgia causes knots in the muscles that can be felt. These localized spasms feel firm, hard and bumpy and you can use your sense of touch to appreciate this. Goose bumps can be felt. The trick is to be able to touch the muscles in a gentle enough manner so as to feel the spasms, but not to aggravate them. Remember, don't try this on strangers.

Learn how to massage your mate's muscles. Take a couples massage class and discover new treatment and intimacy skills.

**5) Taste sensation.** (No this isn't a prelude to Chapter 12). I don't advise you to taste your significant other, and certainly don't advise you to taste complete strangers to look for fibromyalgia clues. There is nothing to find anyway except skin that tastes like mentholly soap.

Your keen senses will make a good fibromyalgia team scout. Search for an understanding of this game. Go to the doctor with your significant other, or to seminars. I like when a significant other comes with the patient to see me; it shows commitment that is much appreciated. Read about fibromyalgia on your own, or whatever she/he asks you to read. Make knowledgeable comments to show that you are fibro-intelligent.

You need to identify bad days, not just the obvious – when she/he looks bad and screams at you, but subtle, earlier clues that a bad day is occurring. Notice these clues, these non-verbal signals that you can see, or the statements that you can hear. Heck, learn how to smell clues. A good example of a knowledgeable comment might be "Your eyes look tired, and you are walking slower; you look like you are having more pain today."

Be the kind of scout that never comes back empty-handed. Make your hunter ancestors proud!

# Scoreboard!

1) Look for signs of pain.

2) Listen for complaints.

3) Check with significant other about your colognes or lotions.

4) Learn your significant other's body, explore with massage.

5) Keep a pain log; what aggravates and what helps.

6) Go to the doctor, attend seminars.

7) Explore alternative medicine strategies.

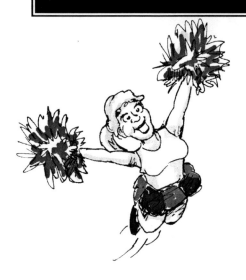

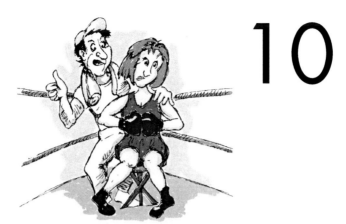

# The Athletic Trainer

Another sport professional that the fibromyalgia supporter is required to be is an Athletic Trainer. An Athletic Trainer handles multiple athletes and needs to know each individual's traits and personality. The Athletic Trainer knows what athletes like to eat, how they train, how they play, and when they need to rest. When anything is wrong, the trainer will know what the problem is and how to fix it.

In fibromyalgia, the Athletic Trainer must learn to handle multiple aspects including fluctuating moods, numerous associated conditions, various interpersonal problems. You need to learn how to feed your significant other who has fibromyalgia.

Your scouting skills will help you recognize and sense the fibromyalgia. Your trainer skills will help you handle the fibromyalgia.

Sometimes you don't know what to expect from your loved one. On good days, all is well and normal, but on bad days, you may be confronted with various moods, emotions, and seemingly different personalities. Your challenge, if you choose to accept it, is to handle all these successfully. Good luck, Jim.

How can you do this? No one really knows. But here are some suggestions for handling different personalities.

Some days your significant other may feel depressed and think negatively. She blames herself for everything. She thinks she is worthless. She expects things to get worse. She is forgetful and thinks she is getting dementia. She has a low self-esteem.

What can you do to handle this personality? You can try dressing up like a Prozac pill, but that probably won't help. The most important thing you can do for her is: connect.

You need to find a way to make a connection with her to let her know that she is not out there all alone; she is connected to the world which you are a part of. Let her know that you are there and that you care about her. She will realize that she must be worth enough to have someone like you care about her. Reassure her that she is a good normal person who happens to have fibromyalgia, and that she is allowed to have bad days, but that you want to help her think positively and feel good about herself.

How do you handle those times when your significant other assumes that perfectionistic role? Everything has to be just right and you can't seem to do anything right, or you certainly are not trusted to do anything the way it should be done. So you don't bother to try because you won't do it right or certainly not as good as your significant other would do it. And if your significant other did not have so much pain, the particular task would get done properly.

You have to recognize that people with fibromyalgia have a perfectionistic and overachieving nature and have a problem handling criticism. They fear losing control, rejection or failure because of the fibromyalgia. They need constant approval.

How do you handle this perfectionistic personality?

---

Try to get your significant other to focus on the positive outcomes of his/her perfectionistic nature. That is, your significant other is very good at being organized and efficient, responsible, reliable, and trustworthy.

Help your partner tell you what main goal or outcome is expected. For example, if you have agreed to get groceries, find out the most important components of getting the groceries. Are there certain items that need to be prioritized, can there be any substitutes, can additional items be purchased? Have your loved one write a specific list and know what your parameters are. That way you know exactly what is expected even before you start the process of actually buying groceries. There is no way you can make any mistakes, right? Try to get your partner to lower expectations without feeling he or she has failed. (Good luck again, Jim).

Anger is a difficult emotion that frequently surfaces in the person with fibromyalgia. The anger is directed at the fibromyalgia and usually is in conjunction with questions like "Why me, I can't do these things anymore; nobody understands what it's like," etc. Anger can lead to negative and destructive consequences in relationships, and within the individual. Anger creates increased stress in the body which can cause more medical problems.

Anger is not right or wrong. It is an emotion and you need to find the right place to put it.

When this angry personality surfaces, encourage your partner to find a constructive outlet for this anger. Acceptable outlets include venting, hitting a punching bag or a pillow, pacing, fast walking, playing a musical instrument, talking to telephone solicitors, and more.

One patient of mine said that she would watch an action-packed movie where the good guys get the bad guys, or play a video game in which you get to shoot things and blow them up. Another patient would go into a quiet forest and scream at the top of her lungs. Anger was channeled out of the body in an acceptable way, although I heard the squirrels were pretty unhappy.

One couple told me when they both get angry or frustrated at the same time, he walks away and she follows him and keeps yelling. They realize it's crazy but can laugh afterwards and say it was good exercise. Try to defuse the situation and see what the real reason is for the anger.

Timeliness is a golden rule for people with fibromyalgia. Being on time seems to be the First Commandment of fibromyalgia. We simply do not know how to handle people who are chronically late. There is a wiring system in our bodies that recognizes time and lets us know if we are on time. If we are not on time, this delicate wiring system signals the heart rate to accelerate, the blood pressure to rise, the sweat to begin dripping, and the anxiety level to magnify tenfold. We simply cannot help it. It is in our nerves.

The best ways to handle the acute attacks of the timeliness personalities, and the safest way if I may add, is to plan to be on time. If you and your significant other are going to some type of social event, mentally plan that this event is actually starting 15 minutes earlier than the invitation says. Once this mental process occurs, you must physically follow through with this reset mental time thermostat and be ready to leave.

One guy I knew tried to encourage his spouse to be more tolerant of tardiness and even practice being late. I hear he's doing better now and she may let him come back home soon!

Another personality trait is a sense of responsibility. The person with fibromyalgia will feel the need to make sure that everything is taken care of for everybody else, usually at the expense of your significant other. For example, a woman with fibromyalgia will feel a responsibility to be the perfect mother, the perfect wife, the perfect best friend, the perfect committee chairperson, the perfect charitable contributor, the perfect volunteer at school, etc. etc. Get the picture? If responsibility were measured in hours, your partner would feel that she/he has 26 hours of responsibility every day.

This responsible personality needs a lot of gentle redirection. Help your significant other recognize that it is possible to be good at a lot of things without solving all the world's problems. Keep reminding your partner that her/his first responsibility is to herself/himself. Try to get the best control of the fibromyalgia. That means prioritizing responsibilities and not taking on new ones, since it is a struggle to do the "old" ones.

Your goal as a supporter is not to take on all of your mate's responsibilities; otherwise, before you know it, you'll have 100 things to do yourself. Rather, your significant other should try to remove responsibilities and just keep the necessary ones that she or he can handle. This might be a rough confrontation because the fibromyalgia person may feel this "letting go" process is a defeat rather than a healthy balance.

Stress is a common personality intrusion. Some days your significant other simply feels overwhelmed, anxious, and literally all stressed-out. Fibromyalgia causes chronic stress in a person. Pretend that there is a lion outside looking at you and trying to get through the window. You see the lion and your body's level of adrenaline and cortisol increases because of the stress. If the lion never leaves, you are under constant tension and this chronic stress can have negative effects on your body over time.

Your job is to help her/him take a stress time-out and

learn how to relax. (You still there, Jim?) There are various ways to achieve relaxation. Both of you can work together to find mutually enjoyable relaxation activities. Examples of ways to achieve relaxation include performing a regular exercise program, taking up fun hobbies, enjoying a hot tub, writing, music, dancing and religion. Stress time-outs should be encouraged daily; schedule them!

Your partner may develop a sense of dependency at times. There may be an urgent sense of inability to do anything without you, or inability to make decisions, or the need for help with all physical activities. This personality trait is certainly undesired as it prevents your partner from being an independent, motivated person who tries to do the most possible in spite of fibromyalgia and its pain. Your role is to provide lots of gentle encouragement. Sometimes you have to set limits on what you are able to help with, and what you expect your significant other to do.

A successful trainer is not trying to change the person with fibromyalgia. Remember you like this person and the fibromyalgia just happens to be a part of the whole person. The trainer's job is to "retrain" the person to use all the skills at the best level.

(Trust me, Jim! Even though you haven't got a prayer in saying or doing the right thing every time, you can learn. Over time, through trial and error, you will help her. A warm hug will always diffuse a bad mood better than a cold shoulder.)

# Scoreboard!

1) Make commitment to participate in your significant other's care.

2) Set priorities on what to accomplish.

3) Encourage talking and communication.

4) Exercise together, do a home program together.

5) Be patient during periods of Fibro Fog, it is only temporary.

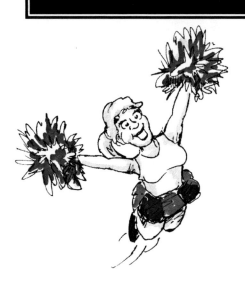

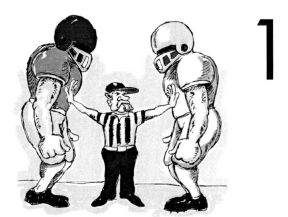

# The Referee

The job of the referee is to try to control the game (fibromyalgia), so rules are followed and it doesn't get out of control. Fibromyalgia will flare up from time to time. Your partner tries to control what she or he can regarding fibromyalgia, but even if all the right things are done, there will still be flare-ups.

A flare-up occurs when there is severe pain and fatigue, more than the usual "baseline." When a flare-up occurs, your partner will experience more pain and fatigue and have more difficulty doing basic activities. Sometimes a flare-up is so overwhelming that either all activities have to be reduced or complete bed rest is needed. You need to know when to stop the clock, when to call a time-out, when to throw the flag, when to assess a penalty and when to resume the game.

If your significant other (if a "she") thinks she is experiencing a flare-up, take her seriously. She knows her body, so listen to her and respect her concerns. Approach the situation promptly by being available and sensitive to her feelings. Communicate your concerns and offer to help out however possible. Sometimes, she won't admit she's not feeling well and will shut you out. You need to coax her out, gently.

Your significant other may have to change some plans because of the increased pain. Canceled dinner plans can upset you, especially if you really wanted to go out. However, your partner has different needs; to take it easy and rest, or perhaps to talk and be helped a little. It may be hard for you to accept that your partner doesn't feel good and thus your plans are affected.

How can you handle this? You try to look for creative solutions that fulfill both of your needs. If you have needs at opposite ends of the spectrum, seek a good compromise. Picking up a restaurant take-out meal and having a relaxing candle-lit dinner at home may be a solution to the canceled dinner date. Buy some fresh flowers, a new robe for her, and rent her favorite video for a comfortable evening at home with her favorite snack food. Quality time can be spent together even in the midst of a flare-up.

When the pain is more severe, your significant other may feel a need for reassurance and might be overwhelmed by everything. Often she is angry because she did all the right things and she still flared-up. You have to know when to back off as well. If she says, "Just leave me alone," that is a good clue that you should back off, right? Wrong! When she says that, you need to be more available and provide gentle reassurance and encouragement.

During a flare-up, your significant other may respond at the extremes of emotion. Remember to be patient and gentle because most of the time this kind of talk is coming from the pain and fatigue and is not the true personality of your significant other. Your significant other needs reassurance and validation of being a worthwhile person.

With fibromyalgia, and particularly during a flare up, your significant other will be seen in a different light. You may not yet be used to seeing the fibromyalgia look: bags under the eyes, pained facial expressions, a frumpy look, the hair in every direction look. It's like that mythical "morning look" that we're asking you to get used to as an "every day look" during a flare up. I advise people not to interpret the fibromyalgia look as negative or bad, but simply as realistic.

I always try to emphasize the positive. Even though your significant other is in a different light, it is still an illuminating light. Your significant other will try to be positively realistic and try to put a positive spin on appearance by dressing up (or at least wearing a stunning bathrobe!), fixing hair, and trying to look as good as possible, even if she/he doesn't feel very well. You could offer to wash and style her hair and give her a pedicure.

The referee is adept at using body language to signal certain game behaviors. Use non-verbal signals to be physically close to your significant other. Make eye contact; have a concerned look. The "open posture" is a non-verbal way of showing concern. In the open posture, you face your significant other a few feet away, have her aligned between your shoulders, make eye contact and avoid crossing your legs away from her or turning your back to her. A gentle touch, a quiet voice, a devoted presence will all be noticed and appreciated.

Help your significant other plan treatments to try to help the flare-ups disappear and return to the base-line state. Patient-directed strategies include using moist heat and muscle creams, taking a hot shower or hot bath, gentle stretches and range of motion. A flare-up may require a doctor-directed strategy such as prescription medicine, trigger point injections, physical therapy, and more. Be part of her treatment plan.

Let others, such as family members, co-workers or chore doers, help out whenever possible. Your significant other may experience a temporary inability to carry out her responsibilities during a flare-up, so use your athletic trainer skills to coordinate various team projects to help out.

There are various ways to maintain a healthy relationship within the support system:

1) **Redefine relationships.** Painful chronic medical conditions can strengthen the bonds between people by letting them focus on the good, positive qualities that made the relationship a good one to begin with. Making a career change (i.e., different job, retiring, work out of home) may be a good decision for the person with fibromyalgia and the support team, and may improve the quality time, quality interactions and happiness and spiritual strength. Mutual respect in each other's roles is very important.

2) **Special get-aways.** Identify places where you can spend relaxing time with your significant other. Consider this your own special place, your retreat, or your oasis in the midst of everything. Plan these retreats to improve your quality one-on-one time, or one-on-family time.

3) **Appreciate the little things.** A phone call, a little note, a compliment, sharing a story, or just being together are mini treasures in themselves within our busy lifestyles. Learn to create and appreciate these positive moments.

4) **Keep your sense of humor.** This is a nice concept that really works. Some of the funniest people I've ever met have fibromyalgia! Since they know the "dark side" already, they appreciate the lighter side even more.

Acknowledge the fibromyalgia and its associated pain, particularly when it is flared up. Bite your tongue if you find yourself ready to blurt out:

> "You have to learn to live with it."

> "It's not that bad."

"I've hurt like that before."

"I know what you're going through."

"You look fine."

"There's nothing wrong."

"Maybe you shouldn't have done that."

Statements like these are very hurtful to the person in pain. They could also result in your head being bitten off!

After the flare-up has settled down and all is calm, go back over the flare-up and review what happened and what may have helped. That way, the next time you can have an active role in helping the flare-up be less of a problem and get it resolved in a shorter period of time.

A successful referee blends into the game and makes the right calls. Unsuccessful referees get booed and booted from the big leagues. Be a good ref; make the right calls and let's try to keep the fibromyalgia person off the injured reserve list.

# Scoreboard!

1) **Learn to identify bad days early.**

2) **Evaluate treatment and find out what works.**

3) **Make quality time for each other.**

4) **Help accept and define limitations.**

5) **Reassure what's going on with the body.**

6) **Be flexible and ready to make alternative plans.**

7) **Learn when to intervene, when to get help from the doctor.**

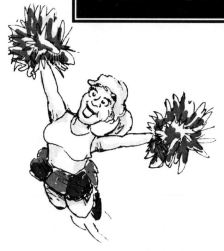

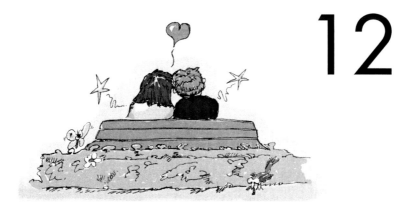

# 12

# Sex and Intimacy in Fibromyalgia (OK, here we go...)

Chronic pain and illness can affect sex and intimacy in a relationship. Fibromyalgia and its chronic pain can intervene and introduce new fears, concerns, and anxieties in a relationship. You may be worried about hurting your significant other during intimate acts. You may feel neglected if the fibromyalgia should lead to decreased responsiveness and frequency of intimacy with your partner.

Your partner, likewise, is dealing with fears and anxieties. Open communication is the most important factor in dealing with sex and intimacy problems.

Fibromyalgia affects everything else, so you shouldn't be surprised that it creates some unique problems regarding sex and intimacy. The main problem is pain, which is the physiological equivalent of a cold shower. Muscles that hurt with pressure and squeezing can "talk louder" during attempts at intimacy.

Many women with fibromyalgia have pelvic pain due to involvement of the low back and pelvic muscles. This can cause painful intercourse.

Men with fibromyalgia may have severe low back

pain with traditional positions during sex. Many patients have reported to me that the muscles may develop a painful cramp right in the middle of intercourse which creates a "major distraction."

Part of the goal is to prevent a statement such as "not tonight, I hurt all over," from becoming too frequent. A better saying might be, "Let's start gently and see where the muscles take us."

Another fibromyalgia-related problem is fatigue. Energy is required to be sexually active, and as I have mentioned earlier, there is very little energy at times with fibromyalgia. Your significant other may be going to bed three hours before you do, so by the time you are ready for bed, your spouse is in the deep sleep stage. This short lived deep sleep stage is highly coveted in fibromyalgia and I guarantee that this deep sleep will be desired more than you at 11:30 p.m.

Another problem related with fibromyalgia is side effects from treatments of fibromyalgia. Specific medicines, particularly those that increase serotonin level (called selective serotonin re-uptake inhibitors) can decrease the sexual response. In women, this means decreased sexual desire or responsiveness, or inability to achieve orgasm. In men, there may be decreased libido or difficulty achieving erections.

Other medicines can cause extreme sedation which prevents sexual alertness. Still other medicines may cause gastrointestinal side effects that focus more attention on the bathroom than the bedroom.

So is it bad to have sex in fibromyalgia? Of course not. Focus on the benefits of sex rather than the problems. Think of sex as therapeutic. For example, this type of physical activity increases the body's endorphins, which are natural pain killers. Many patients state it's the only time they aren't in pain. The physical activity provides stretching, conditioning, and relaxation of the muscles. One tends to forget about pain during intimacy (even if it is only for a few minutes). Being sexually active is a universally "approved" therapy for fibromyalgia (although it is not covered by insurance).

Fibromyalgia does not physiologically interfere with the sexual functions even though there may be some problems because of the pain, fatigue and treatments. You need to be reassured that you are not hurting your partner by becoming intimate; rather you are helping the fibromyalgia and the relationship. Here are some suggestions for having a more satisfying and fulfilling relationship in spite of chronic pain.

**1) Open communication.** Talk to each other and discuss what hurts and what helps, and overcome any fears and anxieties that are present.

**2) Don't poke, squeeze or playfully slap.** It is okay to stroke gently, massage, rediscover touch, and learn the definition of the word "gentle." Take more time to get ready (foreplay ... remember?)

**3) Find comfortable positions.** Certain positions may be painful for the partner with fibromyalgia, but others are not. Positions that involve arching the back, straightening the legs, twisting the spine, or positions requiring a lot of support from only one leg or one arm can be often painful for an individual with fibromyalgia and can lead to muscle cramps. Side-lying positions, lying on the back with knees bent, sitting positions or positions where there may be support on the back may work better. Experiment with different positions. "Rotate" these positions just like one would rotate between sitting, standing and walking at work. Being in one position too long can cause muscle cramps, so be natural but be "shifty" too.

**4) Rediscover the romance.** Touching, hand-holding, kissing, couple's massage and couple's hot tub, can be excellent forms of intimacy. Intimacy does not mean sex alone or having sex at all. (Seriously, look up the definition if you don't believe me).

**5) Redefine what is natural.** Sexual intimacy is natural and needs to felt as such, even if certain things are modified. The physical environment should have a comfortable room temperature without drafts which can increase the muscle pain. The surface should be comfortable. Your partner may need more time and attention to get aroused and should not be approached when physically exhausted. Remember that sexual activity will not damage fibromyalgia muscles, so have fun.

**6) Professional counselling.** Working with a health professional who is experienced in treating problems related to sex and intimacy may be necessary for some couples. It may be difficult to talk about intimate personal problems to each other or even to the doctor. Many physicians and health professionals are skilled and comfortable discussing sexual matters. Through training or professional experience, these professionals can provide valuable insight and recommendation or can refer you to someone who will be able to help you. Counselling is an option.

Remember, underneath the fibromyalgia is still the same person that you love. Showing this love is a mental and an emotional process, not just physical. If fibromyalgia has interfered with this total process of showing love, then you both need to acknowledge this and make a commitment that this interference will only be temporary as you learn to redefine intimacy on your new terms. Don't let fibromyalgia rob you of the pleasure of having it all!

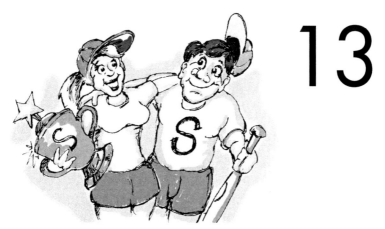

# Becoming Teammates

Relationships can change because of fibromyalgia. Sometimes they change for the worse or even self-destruct.

Relationships include significant others, families, friends and co-workers. Your responsibility is to make your relationship with a loved one who has fibromyalgia as positive as possible.

You can't become teammates overnight. As real-life teammates, you start off almost as total strangers to this new problem of fibromyalgia, then you work with each other and practice skills over and over. At the same time you are improving your individual skills, you are working on a chemistry between the two of you and learning each other's moves, rhythms, strengths and weaknesses. Ultimately, after much hard work, you evolve into your new role as a teammate.

You need to become comfortable with your new role. Your loved one is trying to find the comfort zone with fibromyalgia. He or she may feel guilty on one hand wanting to avoid aggravating the condition, but on the other hand not wanting to neglect your needs. You want to respect your significant other's fibromyalgia and the time required to tend to it, yet you don't want the fibromyalgia to interfere with quality time.

Both of you should become more comfortable at recognizing, communicating and responding to each other's needs. Don't play a guessing game to figure out how each other is feeling at any particular time. Use the clues that you have learned; most importantly, ask, communicate, and connect.

As we get older, we are not the same as we once were. Hardly any of us can do the same things at age fifty that we did when we were twenty. This occurs whether or not we have fibromyalgia, so we can't blame all of our losses on the fibromyalgia.

Likewise, relationships suffer from lack of communication, lack of commitment, lack of self-esteem, complaints about bad habits, nagging, laziness and more, even without the fibromyalgia. So we can't use fibromyalgia as a convenient scapegoat for our problems. Teammates recognize this.

Teammates accept the fibromyalgia. The significant other happens to have fibromyalgia and that's part of the total package now, like it or not. So agree to like it - better yet, love it! You have learned about fibromyalgia and you feel more secure in your knowledge. The next step is to work together to understand and accept the condition and any challenges that may be present.

You want to be positive on redefining the relationship and become ideal partners. You can learn to compliment her/his good and perhaps offset some of the bad that fibromyalgia can bring. You both have always brought your unique perspectives to the relationship, even prior to fibromyalgia. These perspectives have been shaped by both yours and your loved one's past experiences and accomplishments.

Since the diagnosis of fibromyalgia, your past experiences are used to reshape your present and future relationship. Only now you have an additional family member, the fibromyalgia! Like a shadow, the fibromyalgia goes wherever you go in the relationship. You can accept that, but you can also try to have bright sunlight directly over your relationship as much as possible so that this shadow is always small.

There are some rules in enjoying a fulfilling relationship in spite of fibromyalgia:

1. Love unconditionally.
2. Accept fibromyalgia as part of your significant other.
3. Make a commitment to understanding how fibromyalgia affects both of you.
4. Keep a sense of humor.
5. Be grateful and appreciative of your significant other and what she/he is able to do.
6. Enjoy each other whether there is a flare-up or stable baseline.

Communication is always the key in developing a positive relationship. It may be difficult for you to communicate feeling. However, a true teammate will recognize that compassion and sensitivity are necessary to help your loved one hurt less. No matter how tough the game is, always keep talking and connecting.

Married couples took the vow to be together in sickness and in health, for better or for worse. Everyone brings some baggage into a marriage; the married couple makes the best of packing all of this baggage in one suitcase. In the case of fibromyalgia, there is a lot of physical "baggage," whether it came along with the marriage or developed afterwards.

Fibromyalgia can certainly cause sickness and worst

times in a relationship, but a strong foundation of love will allow the teammates to continue playing for a winning team. Teammates may struggle at times at the their positions, or have bad days, but they choose not to let the illness disrupt their solid foundation.

Significant others who are not married have the opportunity to make similar choices on whether the fibromyalgia will come between them. If that ever happens, it does not make them bad people, perhaps just bad at handling the fibromyalgia. Fibromyalgia and other chronic illnesses can cause relationships to end. That is reality. But each person can choose to not let fibromyalgia dominate a relationship. Instead, concentrate on the commitment to be together and love each other in spite of the fibromyalgia.

Just as the person with fibromyalgia has individual needs, so does the supporter. You need to play your position on the team too: Take time for yourself. Don't feel guilty dealing with your own feelings, especially anger or resentment.

The disruptions in your social life (for example, being unable to get out with friends as much) or significant financial change (from loss of job or reduced income) are examples of extreme stresses that can affect your own feeling of well being. Allow yourself time to visit with friends, play a round of golf, go shopping, keep a journal, or confide in someone. Individual quality time will only help you feel more confident and appreciative of your quality time together.

Teammates learn to play the game together. Whether you are shopping, paying bills, traveling, doing household chores, remodeling your house, or exercising, you and your significant other both can plan your work and work your plan. Use your imagination. Plan a getaway and rent a custom van with reclining seats, daybeds and room to stretch. Go shopping during your significant other's best time of day where there is less traffic and crowds. Buy things from a catalog. Throw in a load of laundry and run the vacuum for your significant other. Reorganize cupboards, install a hot tub (for two!), buy each other funny cards or pictures to laugh. Remember to have fun and enjoy each other.

Love conquers all, so demonstrate love. Your loved one's illness provides you with the opportunity to reinforce your love continuously. Your partner is struggling to love this "new self," so make it easier by loving your "new" partner. Your teammate is counting on you.

# Scoreboard!

1) **Recognize that the diagnosis of fibromyalgia is poorly understood and sometimes not accepted.**

2) **Establish confidence in the accurate diagnosis and the body's functioning.**

3) **Develop and show an attitude of tolerance and acceptance towards people with disabilities.**

4) **Say, "I used to think that way before I understood the condition".**

5) **Be an advocate for your significant other and fibromyalgia.**

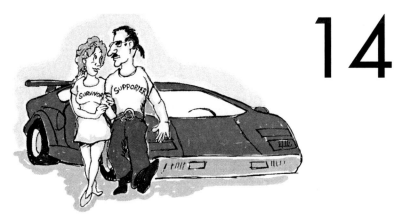

# Fibromyalgia Survivor and Supporter Forever

You and your partner have learned to become ideal teammates forever. Your partner is a fibromyalgia survivor. That means she/he is an active participant in understanding and managing the fibromyalgia. Education, proper body mechanics, medications, exercises, and home program are all part of taking an active role in being a fibromyalgia survivor.

Your significant other accepts fibromyalgia and has learned strategies for best managing it. It is an ongoing effort and enables better control over the fibromyalgia as time passes.

As the fibromyalgia supporter, you too have learned strategies for managing your significant other's fibromyalgia. You have learned how the condition affects you as well as your loved one, and you have accepted the fibromyalgia. You both work hard towards a fulfilling relationship together.

As a fibromyalgia supporter, you continue to evolve into a person who is compassionate, trusting, sensitive, concerned and thoughtful. You have learned to communicate with your partner and encourage her or him to achieve the fullest potential. You have become an enabler, both through conscious effort and practice, and some of it "just happened." All of this was possible because of love and commitment.

You have learned to appreciate a stable baseline of pain. However, when the pain worsens and there is a full-blown flare-up, you will be able to call upon all your resources and tricks, (your athletic skills) to help your loved one through this difficult time.

You have found the balance - physical, mental, emotional and spiritual - and you both can draw strength from each other. Sometimes the balance shifts a little but you have a built in self correcting system that works.

You can believe you both will have better control over the fibromyalgia as time passes, and the flare-ups become less frequent or less bothersome, or more quickly relieved. You will survive the flare-ups together, because you have made responsible decisions and lifestyle changes. You've both committed to maintaining the highest qualify of life together as possible.

As you grow old together as fibromyalgia supporter and fibromyalgia survivor, you will be able to look back at all your shared moments and treasured experiences and appreciate them. All experiences, whether positive, negative, silly, or sensual, add richness and depth to each relationship and make it unique.

With fibromyalgia you want the relationship to feel like a warm comfortable blanket, secure and satisfying. And when all is said and done, the greatest thing you can do is turn to your partner and say, "I love you and your fibromyalgia."

# Index

## A

accepting supporter . . . . . . . . . . . . . . . . . . . . . . .38
adenosine triphosphate . . . . . . . . . . . . . . . . . . .18
aging star . . . . . . . . . . . . . . . . . . . . . . . . . . . . .36
allergies . . . . . . . . . . . . . . . . . . . . . . . . . . . . . .25
anger . . . . . . . . . . . . . . . . . . .27, 40, 51, 52, 67, 70
anxieties . . . . . . . . . . . . . . . . . . . . . . . . . . . .63, 65
anxiety disorder . . . . . . . . . . . . . . . . . . . . . . . .25
approval . . . . . . . . . . . . . . . . . . . . . . . . . . . . . .50
athletic trainer . . . . . . . . . . . . . . . . . .40, 41, 49, 60
ATP . . . . . . . . . . . . . . . . . . . . . . . . . . . . . . . . .18
autonomic nervous system . . . . . . . . . . . . . . . . .18

## B

balance . . . . . . . . . . . . . . . . . . . . . . . . . . . . . . .74
baseline . . . . . . . . . . . . . . . . . . . .27, 57, 59, 69, 74
blood pressure . . . . . . . . . . . . . . . . . . . . .23, 32, 52
brain . . . . . . . . . . . . . .12, 18, 20, 21, 22, 23, 24, 32
brain drain . . . . . . . . . . . . . . . . . . . . . . . . . . . . .18

## C

cancer . . . . . . . . . . . . . . . . . . . . . . . . . . . . . . . .26
chest pain . . . . . . . . . . . . . . . . . . . . . . . . . . . . . .25
chronic .9, 13, 14, 19, 27, 33, 36, 37, 39, 44, 52, 53,
            60, 61, 63, 65, 70
coach . . . . . . . . . . . . . . . . . . . . . . . . . . . . .37, 38
cognition . . . . . . . . . . . . . . . . . . . . . . . . . . . . . .21
communication . . . . . . . . . . . .11, 38, 63, 65, 68, 69
complaints . . . . . . . . . . . . . . .1, 26, 29, 31, 44, 68
complement . . . . . . . . . . . . . . . . . . . . . . . . . . . .38
compromise . . . . . . . . . . . . . . . . . . . . . . . . . . . .58
concentration . . . . . . . . . . . . . . . . . . . . . . . .18, 22
connection . . . . . . . . . . . . . . . . . . . . . . . . . . . . .50
constant pain . . . . . . . . . . . . . . . . . . . . . . . . . . .19
constipation . . . . . . . . . . . . . . . . . . . . . . . . . . . .25
coping mechanism . . . . . . . . . . . . . . . . . . . . . . .37
corpus callosum . . . . . . . . . . . . . . . . . . . . . .23, 24
counselling . . . . . . . . . . . . . . . . . . . . . . . . . . . . .66
criticism . . . . . . . . . . . . . . . . . . . . . . . . . . . . . .50
cure . . . . . . . . . . . .4, 8, 9, 32, 37, 38, 39, 40, 68, 74

# D

denial . . . . . . . . . . . . . . . . . . . . . . . . . . . . . . . .37
dependency . . . . . . . . . . . . . . . . . . . . . . . . . . . .54
depression . . . . . . . . . . . . . . . . . . . . . . . . . .18, 27
diagnosis . . . . . . . . . . . . . . . . . . . . .29, 31, 32, 69
diarrhea . . . . . . . . . . . . . . . . . . . . . . . . . . . . . . .25
disease . . . . . . . . . . . . . . . . . . . . . . . . . .3, 26, 39
dizziness . . . . . . . . . . . . . . . . . . . . . . . . . . . . . .25
dry eyes . . . . . . . . . . . . . . . . . . . . . . . . . . .25, 26
dysfunctional . . . . . . . . . . . . . . . . . . . . . .12, 23, 32

# E

education . . . . . . . . . . . . . . . . . . . . . . . . . . .32, 73
emotions . . . . . . . . . . . . . . . . . . . . . . . . . . .23, 49
enabler . . . . . . . . . . . . . . . . . . . . . . . . . . . . . . .74
encouraging supporter . . . . . . . . . . . . . . . . . . . .37
endorphins . . . . . . . . . . . . . . . . . . . . . . . . . . . . .64
energy . . . . . . . . . . . . . . . . . . .17, 18, 19, 20, 32, 64
expectations . . . . . . . . . . . . . . . . . . . . .12, 37, 38, 51

# F

fatigue 3, 7, 14, 17, 18, 19, 20, 24, 26, 57, 58, 64, 65
fear . . . . . . . . . . . . . . . . . . . . . . .14, 37, 50, 63, 65
fibro-fog . . . . . . . . . . . . . . . . . . . . . . . . . . .21, 22
fibromyalgia . . 1, 2, 3, 4, 5, 7, 8, 9, 12, 13, 14, 17,
                 18, 19, 20, 21, 22, 23, 24, 25, 26, 27,
                 28, 29, 30, 31, 32, 33, 35, 36, 37, 38,
                 39, 40, 41, 43, 44, 45, 46, 49, 50, 51,
                 52, 53, 54, 57, 58, 59, 60, 61, 63, 64,
                 65, 66, 67, 68, 69, 70, 73, 74
fibromyalgia supporter . . . 2, 5, 22, 36, 38, 41, 46, 73,
                 74
fibrositis . . . . . . . . . . . . . . . . . . . . . . . . . . . . . . .7
fibrous tissue . . . . . . . . . . . . . . . . . . . . . . . . . . . .7
flare-up . . . . . . . . .28, 39, 40, 57, 58, 59, 61, 69, 74
flare-ups . . . . . . . . . . . . . . . . . .39, 40, 57, 59, 74
free agent . . . . . . . . . . . . . . . . . . . . . . . . . . . . .36
frustration . . . . . . . . . . . . . . . . . . . . . . . . . .27, 37
function . . . . . . .8, 11, 12, 21, 23, 24, 25, 32, 41, 65

# G

get-aways . . . . . . . . . . . . . . . . . . . . . . . . . . . . . .60
goal . . . . . . . . . . . . . . . . . . . .32, 33, 36, 51, 53, 64
golden rule . . . . . . . . . . . . . . . . . . . . . . . . . . . . .52

# H

headaches . . . . . . . . . . . . . . . . . . . . . . . . . . .25, 26
hearing sense . . . . . . . . . . . . . . . . . . . . . . . . . . .44
home program . . . . . . . . . . . . . . . . . . . . . . .33, 73
hormonal problems . . . . . . . . . . . . . . . . . . . . . .19
hormone . . . . . . . . . . . . . . . . . . . .4, 18, 19, 22, 32
housework . . . . . . . . . . . . . . . . . . . . . . . . . . . . .27
humor . . . . . . . . . . . . . . . . . . . . . . . . . . . . .60, 69
hypothalamus . . . . . . . . . . . . . . . . . . . . . . . . . .23

# I

impatient supporter . . . . . . . . . . . . . . . . . . . . . .37
incapacitated . . . . . . . . . . . . . . . . . . . . . . . . . . .13
infection . . . . . . . . . . . . . . . . . . . . . . . . . . . .14, 39
inflammation . . . . . . . . . . . . . . . . . . . . .7, 14, 31
intercourse . . . . . . . . . . . . . . . . . . . . . . . . . .63, 64
intimacy . . . . . . . . . . . . . . . . . . . .45, 61, 63, 65, 66
invisible condition . . . . . . . . . . . . . . . . . . . . . . . .8
irritable bowel . . . . . . . . . . . . . . . . . . .4, 25, 26, 44

# J

jaw pain . . . . . . . . . . . . . . . . . . . . . . . . . . . . . . .25

# L

limbic system . . . . . . . . . . . . . . . . . . . . . . . . . .23
lotion . . . . . . . . . . . . . . . . . . . . . . . . . . . . . . . . .44
love . 2, 9, 13, 14, 27, 33, 34, 36, 40, 49, 51, 66, 67,
        68, 69, 70, 71, 73, 74

# M

massage . . . . . . . . . . . . . . . . . . . . . . . . . .33, 45, 65
medical condition . . . . . . . . . . . . . . . . . . . .3, 8, 60
memory . . . . . . . . . . . . . . . . . . . . . . . . . . . . . . .21
menstrual cycle . . . . . . . . . . . . . . . . . . . . . . . . .13
metabolism . . . . . . . . . . . . . . . . . . . . . . . .19, 26, 27

mitral valve prolapse . . . . . . . . . . . . . . . . . . . . . .25
moist heat . . . . . . . . . . . . . . . . . . . . . . . . . .33, 59
moods . . . . . . . . . . . . . . . . . . . . . . . . . . . . . . .49
movement . . . . . . . . . . . . . . . . . . . . . . . . . . . .19
muscle(s) 3, 7, 8, 12, 13, 14, 17, 18, 19, 29, 30, 31,
        44, 45, 59, 63, 64, 65, 66

## N
needs . . . . . . . .28, 37, 40, 41, 46, 53, 58, 66, 68, 70
neurotransmitters . . . . . . . . . . . . . . . . . . . . . . . . .12
nodules . . . . . . . . . . . . . . . . . . . . . . . . . . . . . .30
norepinephrine . . . . . . . . . . . . . . . . . . . .22, 23, 32
NSAID . . . . . . . . . . . . . . . . . . . . . . . . . . . . . . .4
numbness . . . . . . . . . . . . . . . . . . . . . . . . . . . . .31

## O
orgasm . . . . . . . . . . . . . . . . . . . . . . . . . . . . . .64
outlet . . . . . . . . . . . . . . . . . . . . . . . . . . . . . . .51
over-eager supporter . . . . . . . . . . . . . . . . . . . . .37
oxygen . . . . . . . . . . . . . . . . . . . . . . . . . . . .19, 32

## P
pain . 1, 2, 3, 4, 7, 8, 9, 11, 12, 13, 14, 18, 19, 20, 22,
        23, 24, 25, 26, 27, 28, 29, 30, 31, 32, 33, 43,
        44, 46, 50, 54, 57, 58, 60, 61, 63, 64, 65, 66, 74
panic attacks . . . . . . . . . . . . . . . . . . . . . . . . . .25
physiatrist . . . . . . . . . . . . . . . . . . . . . . . . . . . . .4
pinched nerves . . . . . . . . . . . . . . . . . . . . . . . . . .31
positions . . . . . . . . . . . . . . . . . . . . . .43, 64, 65, 70
psychological . . . . . . . . . . . . . . . . . . . . . . . . . . .14

## R
realistic expectations . . . . . . . . . . . . . . . . . . . . . .38
reassurance . . . . . . . . . . . . . . . . . . . . . . . . . . . .58
redefine relationships . . . . . . . . . . . . . . . . . . . . .60
referee . . . . . . . . . . . . . . . . . . . .40, 41, 54, 59, 61
relationship . .35, 36, 51, 60, 63, 65, 67, 68, 69, 70,
        73, 74
relaxation . . . . . . . . . . . . . . . . . . . .32, 53, 54, 64
resentment . . . . . . . . . . . . . . . . . . . . . . . . . . . . .70
respect . . . . . . . . . . . . . . . . . . . . . . . . .57, 60, 68
responsibility . . . . . . . . . . . . . . . . . . . . . .52, 53, 67

---

romance .................................. .65
Rookie .................................. .37

## S

sedation ............................... ..64
self-esteem ......................... ... 50, 68
sense ....... .21, 27, 43, 44, 45, 49, 52, 54, 60, 69
sensitivity ............................14, 69
serotonin ..................... .18, 22, 32, 64
sex ..................... .35, 61, 63, 64, 65, 66
significant other. .1, 5, 14, 17, 22, 26, 27, 30, 35, 39,
              40, 41, 44, 45, 49, 50, 51, 52, 53,
              54, 57, 58, 59, 60, 63, 64, 67, 68,
              69, 70, 71, 73
signs ................................. .43
skills ........... .2, 36, 37, 45, 49, 54, 60, 67, 74
skin ...................... .12, 13, 18, 44, 45
sleep ........... .7, 18, 19, 21, 23, 25, 26, 32, 64
smelling sense ......................... .44
spasms ......................... .30, 31, 45
SSRI ................................. .4
stomach cramps ........................ .25
stress ..... .14, 17, 22, 27, 28, 36, 39, 51, 53, 54, 70
stretches .......................... .33, 59
substance P ......................... .4, 32
supporter . .2, 5, 22, 36, 37, 38, 40, 41, 46, 53, 70, 73,
         74
symptoms ..................... .7, 24, 26, 28

## T

taste sensation ......................... .45
team scout ...................... ..40, 41, 45
teammate ............... .38, 67, 69, 70, 71, 73
tender point(s) ........... .3, 7, 14, 26, 29, 30, 31
therapy ..................... .4, 33, 39, 59, 65
tilt table ............................. .32
timeliness ............................ .52
tissues ...................... .7, 12, 18
TMJ ................................. .25
touch sense .......................... .45
touching ............................. ..65
trainer .................. .40, 41, 46, 49, 54, 60
trauma ............................... .3, 14

treatment . . . . . . .12, 26, 32, 33, 37, 45, 59, 64, 65
trigger point injections . . . . . . . . . . . . . . . . . . . . .59

## V
visual sense . . . . . . . . . . . . . . . . . . . . . . . . . . . . . .43

## W
weather . . . . . . . . . . . . . . . . . . . . . .27, 37, 39, 44
weight . . . . . . . . . . . . . . . . . . . . . . . . . .26, 27, 39

# More Ways for "Helping You Live Life to the Fullest"

If you enjoyed *The Fibromyalgia Supporter*, you will be interested in other resources from Anadem Publishing. Anadem Publishing is devoted to providing health information to assist patients with chronic conditions in taking charge of their recovery and in getting the most out of life.

### Fibromyalgia – Managing the Pain
*by Mark J. Pellegrino, M.D.*

Dr. Pellegrino delivers a comprehensive guide to the syndrome. It is the ideal book for the recently diagnosed FMS patient from the doctor whose treats fibromyalgia patients and has it himself.

### The Fibromyalgia Survivor
*by Mark J. Pellegrino, M.D.*

The *Fibromyalgia Survivor* is packed with good advice and tips on every aspect of living your life to the fullest. You get the specific step-by-step "how to's" for daily living. Plus, you learn Fibronomics, the four key principles that help you minimize your pain in every situation.

### Understanding Post-Traumatic Fibromyalgia
*by Mark J. Pellegrino, M.D.*

Everyone with post-traumatic fibromyalgia will benefit from the reading the first book focusing exclusively on this condition.

### Laugh at Your Muscles
*by Mark J. Pellegrino, M.D.*

An easy, light read that you can enjoy and benefit from.

### Chronic Fatigue Syndrome: Charting Your Course to Recovery
*by Mary E. O'Brien, M.D.*

Mary O'Brien, M.D., shares her personal experience in overcoming many of the debilitating effects of Chronic Fatigue Syndrome. In an easy-to-read, nonmechanical format. Dr. O'Brien shares advice on treatment options and self-help steps that will help you rebuild your stamina.

### TMJ – Its Many Faces
*by Wesley Shankland, D.D.S., M.S.*

Fibromyalgia patients frequently suffer from TMJ disorders and orofacial pain. Dr. Shankland's book is filled with step-by-step instructions on how TMJ, head, neck, and facial pain.

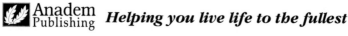 Anadem Publishing    *Helping you live life to the fullest*

# Order Your Books Today!

30 Day Money Back Guarantee
For fastest service, call 1•(800)•633•0055

| Qty | Title | Price (US$) | Ohio Price* | Total |
|---|---|---|---|---|
| | Fibromyalgia:Managing the Pain | $12.45 | $13.17 | |
| | The Fibromyalgia Survivor | $19.50 | $20.62 | |
| | Understanding Post-Traumatic Fibromyalgia | $16.25 | $17.18 | |
| | The Fibromyalgia Supporter | $15.50 | $16.39 | |
| | TMJ – Its Many Faces | $19.50 | $20.62 | |
| | Laugh At Your Muscles | $ 5.95 | $ 6.29 | |
| | CFS – Charting Your Course to Recovery | $14.25 | $15.07 | |

**Shipping and handling**

For 1 book, add $3.50
2–4 books, add $7.00
5–6 books, add $10.00
7+, please call
Priority mail, add $2.50

*Ohio price includes 5.75% state sales tax

**Subtotal**

Add shipping and handling (see chart at left)

**TOTAL**

☐ Enclosed is my check, made payable to Anadem, Inc.
☐ Charge my credit card: ☐ MasterCard   ☐ VISA

Card No. _____ Exp. _____

Signature _____

Name _____

Address _____

City _____ State ____ Zip _____ Phone ( ) _____

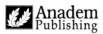

Anadem Publishing   3620 North High Street • Columbus, OH • 43214
1-800-633-0055 • FAX (614) 262-6630
http://www.anadem.com

You can count Anadem Publishing to keep you informed of the newest, most advanced ideas to help you get the most out of life. Let us know if you want to be paced on our mailing list to be notified of new resources. And come visit us at our website! http://www.anadem.com